BATTLE
of a
BORN
Vegetarian

Based on a true story

By M. RAEANN

BATTLE
of a
BORN
Vegetarian

Based on a true story

By M. RAEANN

Copyright©2019
By: Megan R.Ensign

Dedicated To...
Saving the Animals

6

Acknowledgments:

*I would like to Thank **God** for all the plant-life, food-life, and medicine-life he has created and provided for all.*
Then, I would Thank Adolfo Alvarado, the photographer and cover designer.

Table of Contents

A list of Vegetarian or Vegan Greats.....

Pineapple and black olive pizza
Avocado tomato tacos
Fettuccine Alfredo
Banana bread
Mexican rice and beans with fresh tortillas
Sushi
Gumbo and Red Beans and rice
Oatmeal cookies
Peanut butter and jelly sandwiches
Macaroni and cheese
Potato Hominy Soup
Nachos
Cabbage Rolls
Fried Green Tomatoes
BBQ Veggie Skewers
French Toast
Cereal with Almond Milk

12

Introduction

This is a book that consists of true life experiences of the battle and struggles that come along with being a born vegetarian. This life here on earth without meat and poultry, fish, seafood, diary products such as milk. Coming into existence this way is not a choice. It is natural and not have to be focused on or consciously thought about all the time, unless someone else brings it to attention of course.

From the age of four till now in my late thirty's it is the only life I have known. Then later on in life now turned vegan a for the rest of my days.

There are a lot of pros that come with the herbivore lifestyle. There are also a lot of cons that come with it as well. Like the yin and yang, it is like balance to everything. Even our human choice to be a herbivore or carnivore is really a choice.

Most people just thing about the pros of it and do it because of a choice to try something new or gaze into a new lifestyle briefly. To say that they were actually successful at trying something new for whatever personal reasoning. it is great.

There are many reasons for in which people do the things they do. If us as humans did not have to eat to live, then it wouldn't even make something to explain.

In this world we live in and as social creatures, food is a daily talked about issue. So if your habits are not like everyone else then people are curious about a life of living that they could never imagine doing or living.

What we eat and put in our bodies is very important for our mind, body and spirit. So there are people that were actual born a non-meat eater, and at a young age they could not express that it is going to be their way of life. In that young mentality they may not even knowing the reasoning or how to explain it to an adult.

As for being taught to not talk back or say no to adult as a little kid, this can be a very challenging time. Dinner time. When we as humans are old enough to actually control our own spirits, that is when we are vocal about the matters such as what we want to eat or not.

It is the natural born way of looking at meat its self, in the raw, or even worse cooked form. The origin of this thinking did not stem from the "Save the Animal" perspective. That comes later in life. As a very young child, it is simply the perception from the sight, sense, preparation in the food, taste, and texture of the actual food.

Later on with growth and knowledge of the world makes it actually worse. This reasoning is because in knowing the ways of world and what human kind has tried to control, in a way that you know, you can add the "Save the Animal" factor in.

Just surface knowing on how the cows, chickens, pigs, and livestock is treated in America? Those hurt souls, are being eaten by the people whom consumed them. One thing is really sad when it comes to save the animals, is it is all up to Humanity. We were granted the caring for all the plants and animals. Since drones have become a reality, they can now show the world just exactly how the livestock is treated so cruelly.

You are what you eat as the saying goes. So ingesting a sad, torture animal soul who can not speak like humans, is going to make a humans mind, body, and soul, happy? And healthy nourished? Maybe that was the unidentifiable factor in rejecting it as a young child from ages of four years old, or at least when the mind can express it.

Battle of a Born Vegetarian

Chapter 1:

Beef in my Macaroni and Cheese

In the land of the Americas' the continents are rich in food. Along the west-coast of North America, it is rich in sea life. King Crab, Salmon, Oysters, Clam Chowder with fresh clams are just to name a few. Fish of all kinds, like Halibut and Blue Herring. Food of all sorts.

All the different ethnicity here have brought there transitional food cuisine to the Great Northwest. This for sure ads to the different categories of food. Such as Chinese, Japanese, India, Cambodian, Thailand, Filipino, Greeks, Russians, Indian from India, just to mention a few. The land is filled with delicious, unique, original, artistic, creative and not to mention beautiful ways of making food. One that is amazing and local, is from the Native Americans, from surrounding tribes, made smoked salmon jerky.

In this country, as Americans, we like to enjoy a food cuisine called macaroni and cheese. As a five year old that is an awesome dish of food to have. It actually became my favorite. All American Macaroni and cheese. Bright orange little pasta noodles that was cheesy, creamy, hot and filling. In my mind it was a main dish in my little kid menu. This what most people considered a side dish to go with their meals, such as meat and vegetables.

It starts when I was five, and despised meat with a passion. Meat of all kinds and sorts. Absolutely no pork, beef, or lamb, hot dogs, rabbit, venison, elk stew, liver. Never. It was so creepy. It had juices, and worst of all it used to be an animal. In these instances, this is not a stylish, fashionable, trendy, or trying something new type of thing. In this case it is a natural born way of life. This book can explain from the perspective from a lifelong non-meat eater.

There was something about the texture of it. This look was horrifying too. Now you can at all not overlook it and try to distinguish its origin. Most of the meat has been processed, cooked, sauced, seasoned, smoked, prepare and stuffed with stuff. I mean really, that is doesn't sound natural to me. The look it reminded me of the scene from the eighties movie, Yes, it is cheezy, but when the steak started moving on the counter all by itself in front of the person, it was crazy.

It was one afternoon, and we were outside playing. My sibling and I were five and in kindergarten. In our back yard there was an amazing tree house that was build for us. There was a ladder that went from the ground up to the tree house through the floor. It had siding on it and was painted to match the house. In the back of the tree-house as a window that faced the hay field behind our house. As lunch was called we ran in the house, washed our hands and sat at the table. Our parents were gone, and we had a babysitter that day.

In bowls being sat down in front of us the babysitter gave us our lunch. In the bowl was Macaroni and cheese. Yes, I thought. My favorite lunch. Then I zoomed in to the bowl closer seeing my mac an cheese did not at all look the same as it always did.

I asked the babysitter, "Um-mm, what is this"? She responded in a slow, surprised tone of voice with, "Oh that is my mac and cheese with hamburger in it".

Right then, my whole self changed and got sad. I responded with, "I will not eat that, I despise meat". "Do Not take it personal I expressed." Then sharing the feeling with her that the meat had ruined my mac and cheese. At that point I knew I was going to be a strict lifelong non meat eater. The feeling was so strong that I was willing to be hungry if they would not understand.

Another time recalling at the elementary age, there was a box of powdered milk in our food pantry, not to mention a bizarre thing.

So as I was dishing up cereal super fast, because we were going to be late for the bus. As I dumped the powdered milk in my bowl, cereal and added the water, mix it up really quick and couldn't wait to take a bite.

All the sudden in my middle of eating the cereal was balls and lumps of sour powder milk up in the mix of my breakfast. The powder milk it self not mixed was sour, and warm and so gross.

Never again did I want to see powder milk.

Chapter 2:

Timer Goes Off

It was a typical evening for dinner and the course consisted of a hamburger patty cooked with a side of ketchup. There was some random side but my mind was to boggled by the beef patty that I could not remember anything else. As we were dished up, my sibling and I sat at the countertop in the kitchen side by side and looked at our plates.

Immediately, my sibling started cutting the patty with his fork and knife, then proceeding to dip the piece on his fork into the pile of ketchup. I thought oh my gosh, I am for sure not doing that.

At that point the decision was so easy. I then slowly ate whatever side dish that was on the plate. As my sibling grubbed down their plate of dinner, they jumped of the bar stool after looking at me with a face of empathy.

Our caretaker at the time walked into the kitchen and asked me, "Are you going to eat that?"

I responded with, "No way, I do not want to eat this". Like in the children's book Dr. Seuss, Green Eggs and Ham. With that, then she set the timer on the oven at thirty minutes, telling me to finish or I will be going to bed without dinner.

As I sat their at the counter, looking at the timer ticking away, then looking down at the cold, brown, weird looking circle, of non chew-able, no flavor, and rubbery substance that was making me gag. It seemed as if time was slowed down, just because I was being forced to sit there. Well I was going to endure this timing ticking session no matter what.

So the DING sound went off and a second later the caretaker entered the room, looked at the stove, then looked at my plate and saw the cold, shriveled up, nasty, dark brown, Frisbee looking circular pile of unknown substance next to its untouched partner, the pile of ketchup. Out the window with the ketchup too. Never will I, or ever would eat it. They are partners with the hamburger patty.

She then looked up at me and said, "OK, off to bed". Relieved finally, I jumped off the counter stool and ran to my room. Yay.

No more looking that plate of awfulness. As I lay a little hungry, I was happy I was not forced to eat it. The result of that would have been not in the best interest of the adult in charge at the time. They would have ended up cleaning up my getting sick with it.

As morning came, I was excited to breakfast and rushing to the kitchen there was the caretaker standing there saying, "good morning", and she opens the fridge, reaches in and pulls out a plate with the cold hamburger patty from the nightmare night before.

It was unwrapped of plastic wrap and placed on the counter being served as my breakfast.

For not even being awake, and going through an eventful night of kid verses parent, I actually was stunned at the adult.

The fact that they would do such a thing, thinking the child is deliberately acting in rebellion over food. Come on, really? So from that moment on I knew from this point of my five years of age till eighteen was going to be a battle with the adults.

Well to make sure that this timer situation never happened again, my sibling that sat next to me at the counter, well, consider it like them getting second helpings of dinner. Sometimes there was no dinner left for anyone to have seconds, but they got mine. When the adults left the room, or looked away, I sled my meat onto their plate.

In my generation is when the classic movie The Gremlins was released. Now that is a great movie. After see the scene where they trick the kid into letting them eat after midnight, and they way they tear up the plate of chicken legs cold out of the refrigerator, all rowdy, slimy, and sick, my perspective changed as a young child. It made me say to myself, " I will never eat that in my whole life". It just looked wrong even with a Gremlin eating it! Naming these scenes in movies, the humorous part about it, that meat is made scary in scary movies.

That solution solved it all the way around. My sibling got seconds, I didn't have to eat any meat, and sit with timer ticking away, and the parents did not even know. Problem solved.

Chapter 3:

Food Choices

One of the worst things was battling the beef stews in the winter time. When a family actually shot and killed a deer, or elk for the winter to feed thief entire family for the winter, that's literally what they are doing. Eating it all winter long, from being stored in their deep freeze.

Seeing the whole process as a kid was a seasonal normal. From the game being killed, gutted, and sent off for processing, to it coming back in little white wrapped packages that had deer or elk meat. The potatoes and carrots, sometimes maybe corn or green beans, was the savior of the stew.

So the stew was always cooking once a week it seemed. It was a huge kettle type stew pot. The recipe consisted of potatoes, carrots, and the animal meat. In a red saucy type tomato soup. When that soup appeared to be making on the stove, all I could think was, well I am eating potatoes tonight. So today potatoes are a lifeline in my living.

No matter what comedian clowns over your all American potato eating culture well they are just joking and doing their comedic job. When in fact, in South America, Peru, has many different types of potato to eat with different types of meals. This is according to a native Peruvian women who was born and raised their. She was the manager of a Japanese steak house. Also that night she was the cook and entertained us with her culinary expertise with the preparing of our food. She was sharing with us about her country with her accent that was rich and adorable, she had mentioned of over seventy something types of potato in South America, Chile.

As a kid I saw all animals as beautiful, innocent. They are amazing with no verbal communication with humans that belong to God. They are his creatures that reads in the Holy Bible, that he gave them to us humans to care for and look after.

If you think about all the living organisms and life here on earth, its truly miraculous, with all their own intelligent echo systems and reasoning for being here. When they asked you at school what do you want to be when you grow up, well for me my answer was a Veterinarian. Yes, to doctor and help animals.

So in elementary school they had hot lunch, or cold lunch. Our parents signed up us up for hot lunch, because in the winters it was really cold. It was your typical cold day and we were in the lunch line. All the little kids getting their trays of food given to you, off you went to sit and eat. Well sitting there with my second grade classmates, checking out the options on the tray that day. It was some kind of jello, peas and carrots, (canned probably) and for the main course a fried fish rectangle with crusty golden brown crust coating, with a side of tarter sauce.

Everyone thought the fish patty look good, compared other things that were served.

As I grabbed my fork and knife, I cut into the fish patty. It crunched in between my fork., then I opened it in half. I looked and stared at the interior. Something bizarre caught my eye, was it halibut or cod?

I zoomed in and couldn't believe what I was seeing or looking.There were in between my fish patty, white flaky supposed to be fish meat, was different color veins. Yes Veins. Purple ones, and red ones, and light pink ones. I even remember blue ones. It was like a bunch of electrical fibers running through ht the fish meat. Very unnatural looking. In all the times I saw our fresh rainbow trout cut, cleaned in the creek, then grilled, nothing ever looked like that.

I told my classmates, "Hey everyone is there little veins in your fish patties"? Everyone saw my food and was like ,"Gross"!That is disgusting".

From that day on, it was cold lunch, full time. Without a doubt I was going to pack it myself. It was simple, the main course was a peanut butter and jelly sandwich, or instead of jelly, sugar. It was safe for sure. In a little brown happy sack at that.

It was interesting to see the future outlook on hot lunch, and what they were feeding to us not thinking we were paying attention or reject the veined fried fish patties, and cold hamburger meat brown nasty patty on a bun was served!

Chapter 4:

Childhood Vegetarianism

The day to day journey through childhood was going to be eating whatever was there besides the meat dishes was the mission and way of life. The technique of picking out the meat balls in the casserole or picking around the lasagna avoiding the sausage and beef was done in a discrete way. It was a technique done to prevent all from being grossed out at the table or always looking as I messed with my food on the plate, scraping away the meat particles. Many vivid memories flash of scraping gross, cold, sick looking, crumbly, un-chewable, fat, greasy, and brown, or red if raw into the trash. Oh, not to mention, slimy or gooey, like clams, oysters, raw fish, or raw steak.

To some it was called an extreme diet by many, and not a veggie lifestyle. They could not comprehend it, and just stared with a blank stare of nothingness. In the eighty's generation of adults, they had no idea what was going on. So pale and skinny I was considered, or with an eating disorder as the ignorant called it.

A child can not communicate to an adult that they don't like meat and will not eat it at the age of three, or four. This is unless, they are asked, and taught. If not, the child skipping the pig or beef patty is not necessarily showing signs of a extreme eating diet.

One of the joyous memories as a little kid, was looking forward to the weekend for the donuts and candy store adventures. It was the brown bag weekend special.

We were probably only seven years old and on Fridays, we got to take our money and walk about a half mile to the convenience stores.

Before the sun went down we would get ready, grabbed our money and set our on our own. There was a convenience store on either side of the street when we got to the end. At the end was the baptist church we sometimes went to day care there.

On one side was a family run one, and across the street was a commercial one.

Usually we would always go to the family run one. The candy was sold differently and they had boxes that sold candy singly. The little store had a whole section of candy like tootsie rolls, jolly ranchers, gum, pixie sticks, and lemon drops, the best yet was watermelon bubbalicious gum.

Usually we would get a brown bag with candy in it and play at the park on the way home. That bag of candy would last all throughout the week.

Now on Sunday, it was a whole day of another kind of excitement. After the park, but before the convenience stores, there was a little donut shop, next to the post office.Now this donut shop seemed like it was only open on Sundays.

In the morning we would get ready and mostly always would be chilly outside, so we would bundle up. Today we were going to get a brown bag full of freshly baked donuts.

This little donut shop consisted of a little place, with some chairs and a glass case from wall to wall besides the register. It was warm and white inside. To pass by it all the time we would look over and it would be closed. So this Sunday morning it was alive, warm, smelling of donuts. Our parents would give us money less the ten dollars, and we would go get fresh fluffy so good tasting classic donuts. That was an awesome little bakery. The best ones were the apple fritters, and maple bars.

One day arriving home from high school, excited to be out and home and ready to eat and get warm. It was winter and seemed like there was snow all the time up in the pine tree area of the world.

At that point, waking up early enough was nonsense. There was a grip of snow outside in the dark cold. No one wants to be in that verses their warm bed. Before I knew it I would have to be standing out in the snow under the street light all early waiting for the school bus in freezing, icy cold air with a bunch of half awake kids. The sound of silent but nosey snow falling, all nature is asleep, why on earth do kids have to go to school all early in the morning when it is freezing.

So my choice was to skip breakfast, and move right on to school, and lunch was never much, I do not even remember the cafeteria. By the end of the day hunger would set in after thinking all hard from the early morning. There was I ice cream in the freezer what what I was looking forward to.

As I was dishing up the yummy bowl of ice cream a step ex relative my age came down the stairs and said, You can not eat ice cream before dinner". She did not have the luxury of eating ice cream before anytime, so it probably was new to her. Anyways, replying to the controlling spirit, " I can eat ice cream whenever the time I please. "My parent bought the groceries". Shortly after I took my happy bowl downstairs into the basement to grub out, she appears after ,e really to say, "My moms on the phone and wants you to come up to talk to her". My mind raced with so many thoughts I could not even talk. "Like was this real"? It was the only thought that could compute.

I responded with, "You called your mom"? In disbelief, I got on the phone and the mother said, "you need to stay in the basement till we get home".

Chapter 5:

Continuing on to The Adult Battle

It was Friday night and we were in Las Vegas. The lights are so bright, there are sounds going off in all directions. The air was filled with music playing constantly, and everyone is in motion.

The energy is so chaotic that you have to have been there and felt it. Like in a daze, you see a pair of girls arm in arm, with no shoes on just skipping thought the casino on a early Saturday morning, just skipping on air so happy. It is like getting on those floor escalators in the airport, but instead it is an invisible energy force in lanes for walking. Your senses are being stimulated from all directions. It is truly a site to see.

All that can not make you aware of how dehydrated being the desert dry climate, and the physical energy you burn up just having to get to your destinations. Then you ask for a glass of water at a restaurant, and it taste like red, desert, dirt, warm water. So much for quenching your thirst huh? This is without consuming anything but water and coffee, becoming so lacking of water all the time.

All of us got dressed up ready to go to this very pretty restaurant and have a great dinner before a night on the town. Spending time in Vegas can lead to a lot of walking with out being aware of it.

After a day of walking we finally we entering this fancy seafood restaurant, so hungry from exploring the day on our vacation. The atmosphere of the place was dressed in dark wood and white linen clothes on everyone and thing. It had wine collection on the wall and glasses gleaming at each setting. As we sat down we just looked around and admired such a pretty place to eat.

The waiter brought the menus, and considering seafood was not apart of my diet, immediately skimming the vegetable sides menu was where my choices always are.

As the waiter returned we ordered, and all I ordered was a bake potato with everything and roasted asparagus spears. The food was beautiful upon arrive. The presentation of the dinner was nice, and filling. It was peaceful and pleasant.

When the waiter came back, we paid and the person with me mentioned of my vegetarianism. His response was, Oh, well we do have vegetarian menu, I should have brought it". I was wondering why you were eating so light."

So basically, he proceeded to mention the most amazing cauliflower casserole as we were finished and leaving. Maybe in the future all restaurants should mention their meatless menu as well. It could also lead people to look at the menu intrigued getting knowledge of all the different types of dishes. Also it could crush the thinking that vegans eat nothing but lettuce.

I politely thanked him, and said "everything was great". So if your out to eat at a fancy restaurant, I mean this was a five star restaurant we were dining at, ask if they have a veggie menu. Most of the time it might not be offered in the beginning of your setting. If the Vegan Menu would have been offered, ordered way more food is obviously more probable.

It just brought it to light as a actual issue, or conversation for everyone to know at that moment. That is the type of instance were it was made something to talk about, when it is a really personal thing to ones well being.

Let say you get invited to dinner party by someone, and they are throwing the dinner. This means them cooking with their stuff, and menu. When you arrive and are starving ready for dinner, and it ends up all you can eat is the salad. This is where the saying is so very true. Then " Yes, all they eat is lettuce"! That statement was made true probably from these instances. In the case of a dinner party, having to eat before you leave might have to happen.

On the nutrient health side of things being and adult and not getting the mineral iron in red meat, supplements need to be taken in order to prevent anemia. Iron helps the body make red blood cells to help the body and heart run efficiently. As a plant eating person the food that is consumed is important and has to be payed attention too. Almonds are a great source of eating Iron.

Anemia can be a vegetarian based sickness in the blood if it is not taken care of and treated with care. As there are people so obsessed about not eating carbohydrates, or keeping up with their protein intake, well the same kind of attention is needed for the veggie person.

44

Chapter 6:

Denying the BBQ and Save the Animals

There usually is a time during most peoples summer where the BBQ is being cooked. Everyone is gathered in a plain old backyard to water recreation destination that is been awaited and planned for.

The classic menu, for these occasional cookouts, is mainly a carnivorous diet. This consist of any animal that was once alive. Pork, beef, any kind of game. For some reason in this world chicken, fish, and seafood are considered to fall in a different category of our so called human food diet. So they are not the same according to the mainstream one chart for all. So as people are preparing their food, and they take much creativeness in their preparation and culinary skills they are assured for everyone in the mix to enjoy and praise the cook.

Well a lot of time if the steak that just came off the grill is not tried by the non-meat eater, then immediately there is just a little vibe change. Not in all cases, but it has been said, Well, why not try it, it is the best steak ever"! So responding nicely, with I am sure its great and good job but no thank you, their is nothing that could make me try it today, and certainly not tomorrow.

So whatever else is at the BBQ always, either brings your own food, or eat whatever else is on the menu is always the way. No problems, no going hungry. There is so much more to choose from. Like grilled asparagus, avocado taco. Tortilla chips and melted cheese dip. You certainly can not forget the Mexican rice and potato salad or pasta salad. Fruit salad with pecans always makes for a great dessert to add. Not to forget the famous potato salad, or pasta salad. There are the saving with the potatoes and macaroni again! To the rescue.

As an adult now, to know what is really going on in the world makes it easier to be without meat or poultry. With the oil spills and the nuclear spills in the oceans surrounding us is kind of hard to deal with as well.

As the ocean once provided so much, now its empty, sick or full of floating trash. This trash plastic poison part is because of us humans deciding that that is where are going to dispose of the plastic on earth, which is also contributing to the die off of our beautiful sea life. They are being poisoned and dying because humans are catching all their food. Not to mention how good it was to eat twenty years ago, but now you can not compare.

For all the other animals on earth is is sad what humans are doing to them.

From the agriculture stand point being and animal lover it is so hard to see now more than ever how the cattle, and the pigs, chickens, and all others are treated.

The do not have the ability to speak a language to communicate to us, and it does not give humans the right to treat them anyway they want in an inhuman way and it be OK for their million dollar farms. They are sell outs. Killing is Killing. They should really try to do something else, like grow hemp to make toilet paper. Save the trees and the animals. The American President G. Washington grew hemp, and he is on our federal currency. It common sense. So it is a sad situation for the animals. That sad soul is being consumed by who ever eats it.

Chapter 7:

The Nurse and Eating Disorder

Refusing their meat based diet in the hospital for three days the staff put on paper that had an eating disorder was present and needed to be made aware of. Reasoning solely coming from my stay there. Denying and not drink their beef broth, they stated on paper and eating disorder.

There whole menu was gross, and when I didn't partake in their meal time or activity time, they considered it eating disorder like conduct. Which in fact, is a complete lie. After days of not eating their disgusting diet, I had been asking for other food, such as fruit. They never gave it to me.

If the hospital, nurses and staff are so concerned with someone eating to get better, they denied me. In a metropolis at that. We are not even talking about a little medical center or a little town.

Everyday I asked someone for a piece of fruit, and they responded with, "there is none and not going to be any". Instead, they just wanted to shoot me up with sick me medicine, and experiment with Ambian on me.

So even a nurse that works at the hospital can follow you out at your discharge and completely harassed you in the waiting room where no one else can see or hear.

Sitting on the bench anxiously waiting for the elevator to open This little square room. It was the locked, can not leave if you tried doors and then the elevator doors. As I was awaiting on the bench happy to be getting out of this hellhole, she, the nurse of nastiness, proceeds to follow me out and sits next to me on the bench, and no one else around. She leans all close and creepy next to me and proceeds telling me all these lies in my ear. The bull that was being feed to me after I had been starving for days, because the hospital was so broke it could not have a full stock of food.

I denied all their food. It looked so disgusting, worse than jail food. It mostly was beef based, their broth and meals. It made me sick that I had to even go, so I did not want to eat in the first place. Everything was making me sick to my stomach, that it took my appetite completely away. So by this point, I had no time or energy for some bull of nonsense trying to be force-fed to me.

This nurse that was harassing me was telling me on my discharge papers they put an eating disorder and I should see a group of people like a support group or something. I thought," are you crazy?, you are literally making all this up". She was stuttering the whole time, looking at the elevator. She was trying to think of what to say free-styled as fast as she could. You could tell it was hard. Of course its hard to make something from nothing. I remained looking straight ahead and didn't even look at the lady.

My mind was completely shut off from her voice. At that moment, just hearing, like background noise, not listening at all to what she was trying to effect and infect me with, but I turned that nonsense off immediately. I specifically asked them for a banana for two days, and they told me there were none. Knowing that the banana helps with a turning upset stomach and revives with energy. But no, absolutely not one banana in this hospital in a city of one point five million.

The nasty manipulative nurse had no effect on me, except this disbelief in a deceptive human being trying to manipulate.

Chapter 8:

Neighborhood Gardens and Tree Farms.

In all actual reality, if you think about it making a community garden would be great. If every residential neighborhood had a community garden in one of the housing lots, such as next to the community center or around the amenities area. It is disappointing that our past generations did not really set that up for us already in effect full time. The playground was really the necessity.

It could easily be 1ncorporated into the homeowner association yearly fees that include new produce plants and flowers every season. All year around it could be full of fruits, vegetables, trees of the land that produce, and it could have a caretaker, with paid wage and it would be awesome and contributing to the future generations of children.

There are many out there that would love to take care of the food that feeds our neighbourhood, and it allows healthy food for our surrounding neighbors. This could include fresh flower gardens as well, where its OK to go cut a bouquet for you dinner table to go with the beautiful, free, paid for, organic ley grown salad or bowl of fruit on the counter.

An idea of, while the kids are on their walk with their parents, or they are out playing in the playground, they can feel free to go get a snack while they are out is fun. To grab a healthy snack as well. The moms could also cut a fresh bouquet of flowers of the season for their dinning room table as well.

It could also be an educational tool for the children or how to grow food. All this would be at no cost, but the included one in the yearly fee. What would be a way to contribute back is to replant something, or take a little time and tend to the community garden. Even maybe creating a garden, farmers market comity neighborhood community.

The garden could be fenced to keep it safe from the deer or other animals. A greenhouse could also be incorporated as well for the winter time crops. They could also incorporated an herb and spice garden. For example, mint, time, parsley, cilantro, basil, oregano, and more.

The flower garden could be all around the perimeter, such as carnations, and wild flowers, like daises, or sunflowers. This would also help and contribute to the bumblebee population.

There could be a specified day that the community could plant any tree or donate any kind of eatable food or flowers to the garden. They could watch it grow up and produce food for everyone.

The idea of this could be achieved very easily, and create a whole new way for people get food easily whom cant get to the store as easily as others. This could include, the elderly, veterans, people who can not travel far. The list goes on and on. It it really a beneficial thing to many. Once the trees are planted, such as lemons, limes, avocado, and mango in this environmental elements, then after years God willing, they will produce for future generations. Also they could produce more and more every year.

If this were to be done, and a community garden was alive with potatoes, carrots, greens, corn, radishes, squash, tomato, and on and on. There would be trees of all sorts, like avocado, mango, for instance, maybe no one would or any kid would not be hungry and since produce is needed on a weekly basis, is could be easily obtainable in this manor. This concept is to help all with contributing, sharing, saving, caring, and consuming healthy food to bless the body for years and generations to come.

57

The End

Other books by this Author:

God's Power Over Us Part 1
A Miracle in the Night

God's Power Over Us Part 2
A Trip of a Life Time

A Simple Recipe on How to Stop Smoking,
Kick the Habit on Your Own!

www.ingramcontent.com/pod-product-compliance
Lightning Source LLC
Chambersburg PA
CBHW051415250726
48655CB00003B/1072